BREAST CANCER COLORING BOOK

THIS BOOK BELONGS TO

_____

We know that breast cancer is a very serious and sensitive topic. Our mission was to create a book that will help you cope through this difficult time. All quotes were written so that they give a sweary and funnier spin on the concept of cancer. We created this book to help as many breast cancer patients as possible. We want to brighten their day and help them relax their troubled minds. We would like you to know that this was our intention and if you find any of the quotes offensive, please accept our sincerest apologies.

~ Cathy Rose

"I am not afraid of storms, for I am learning how to sail my ship."

~Louisa May Alcott

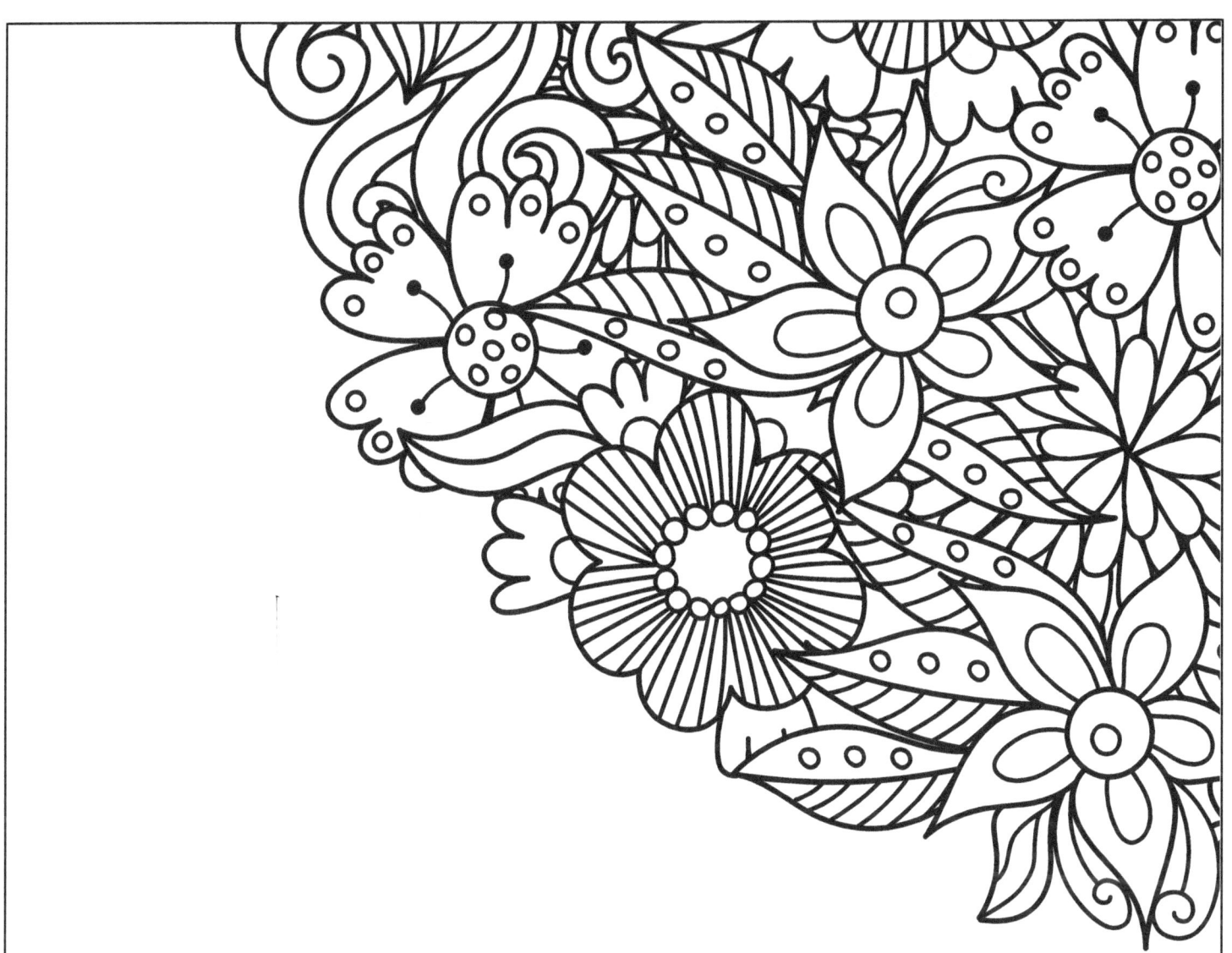

fuck you cancer

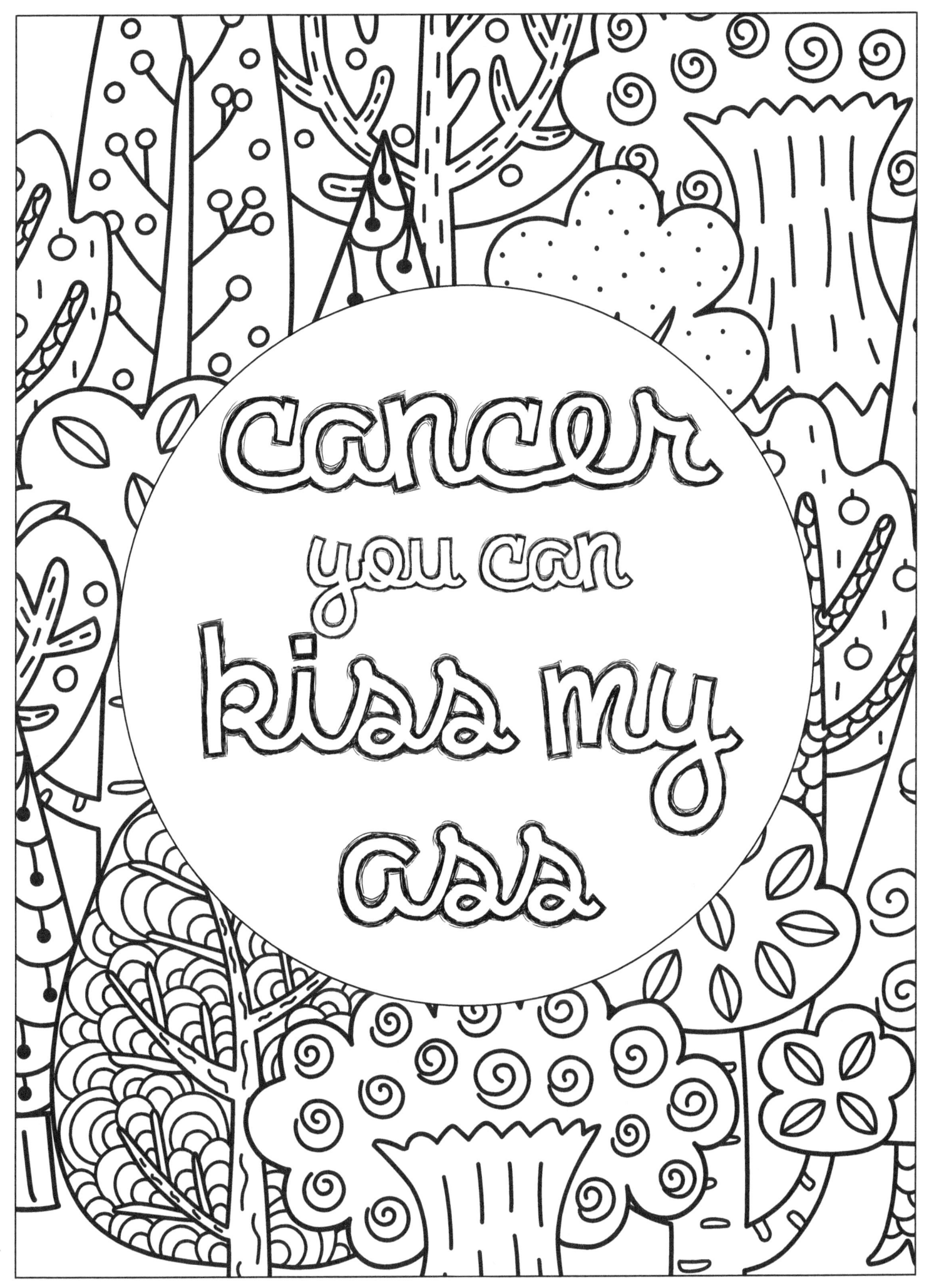

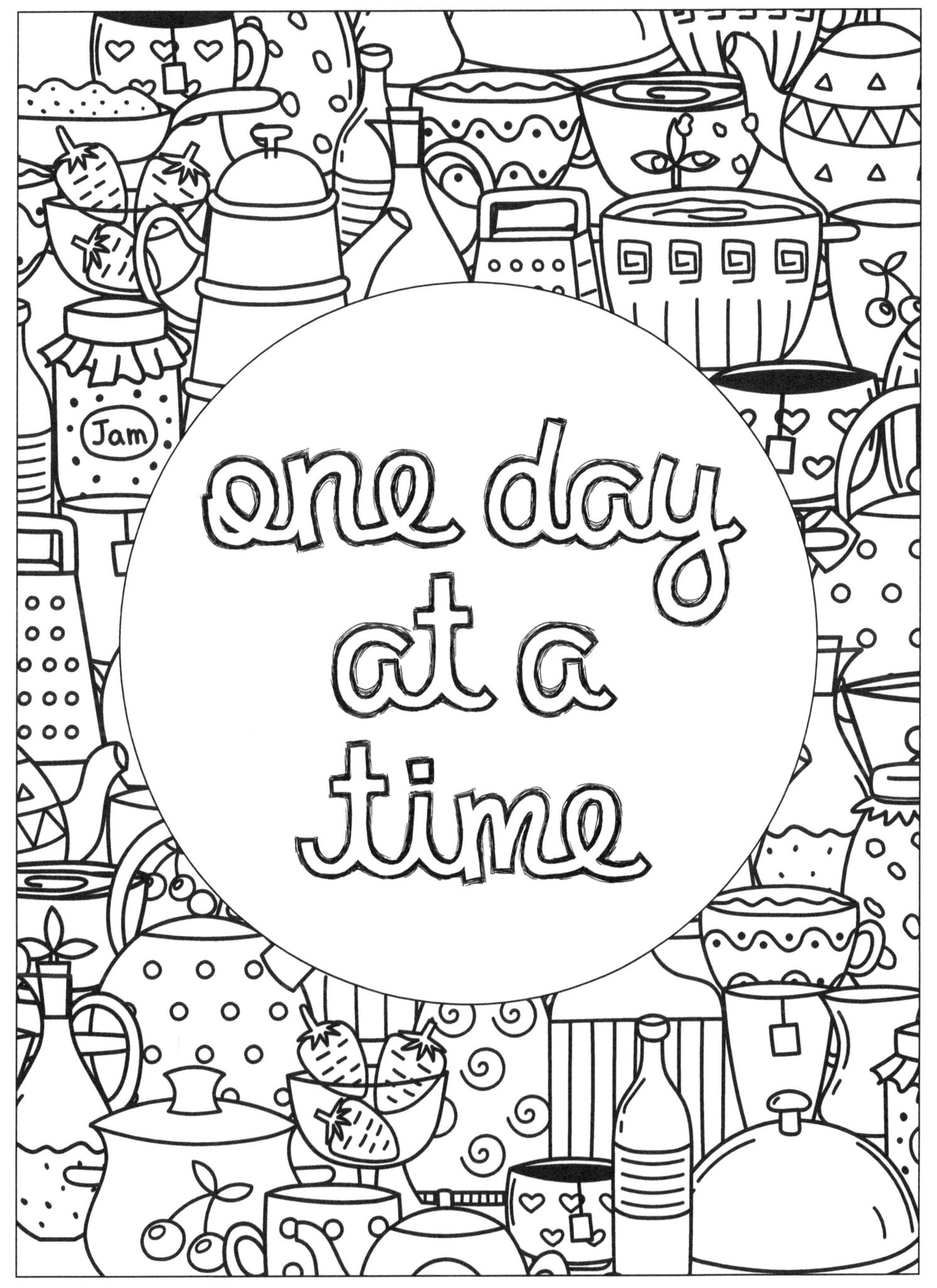

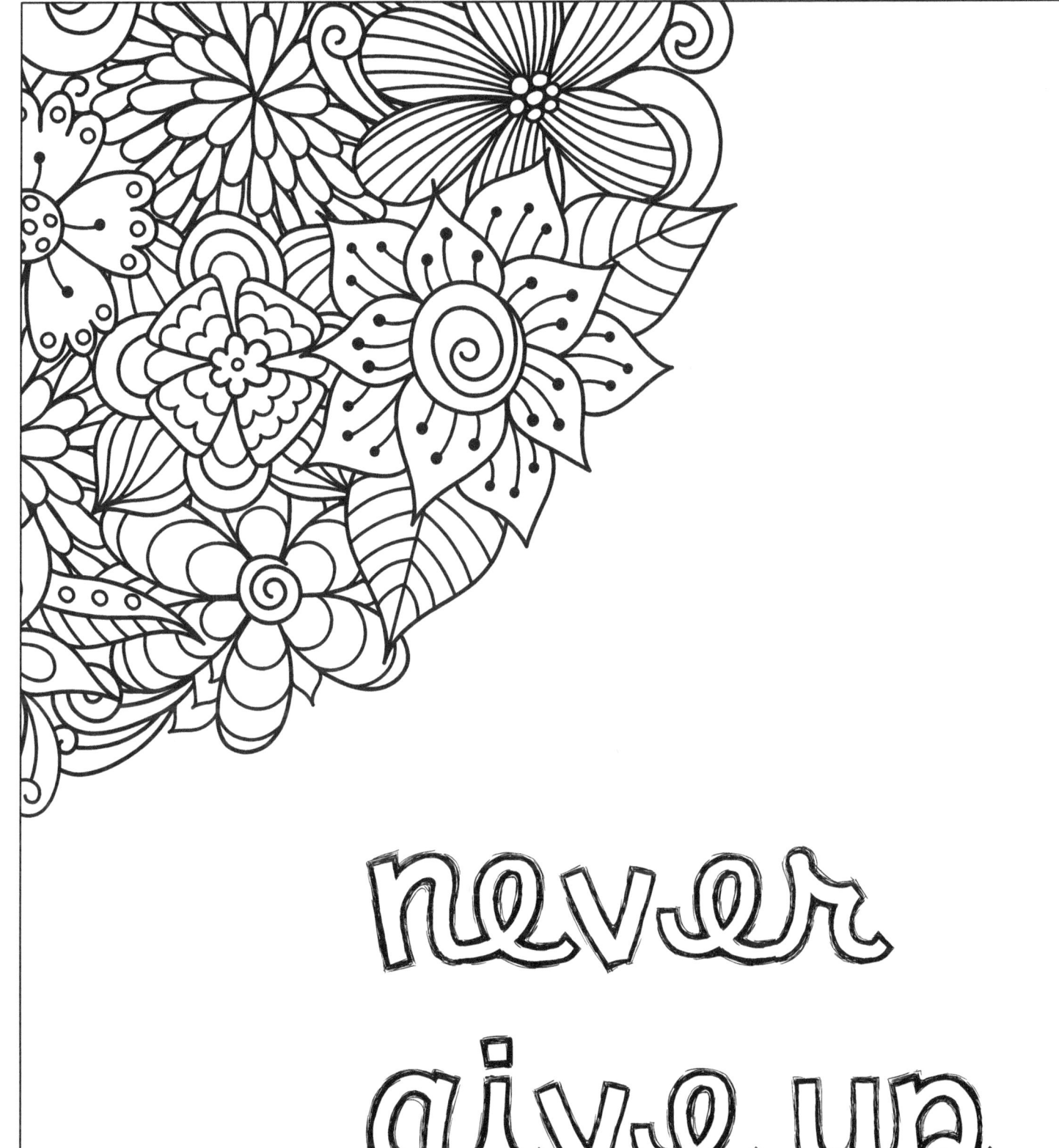

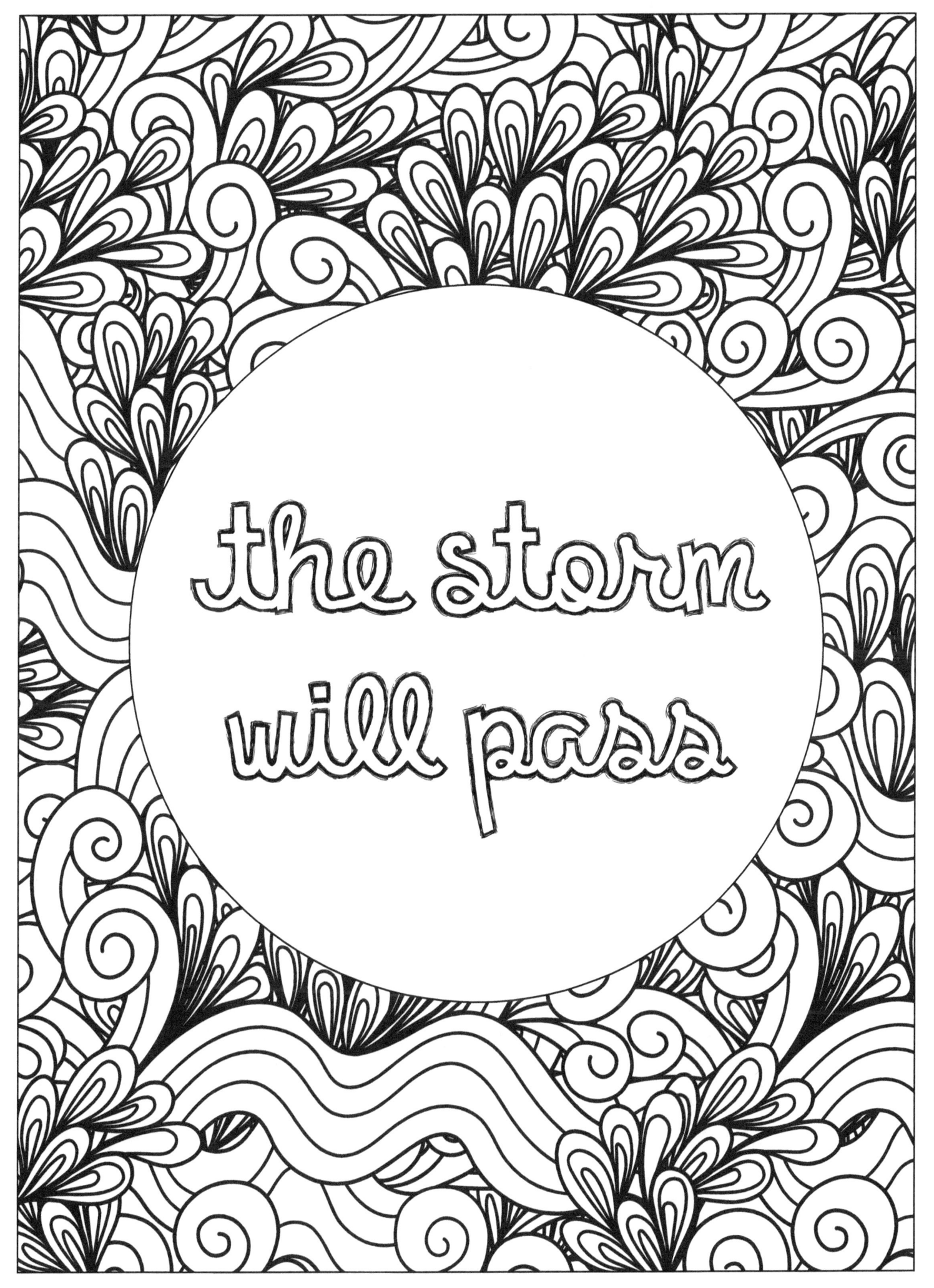

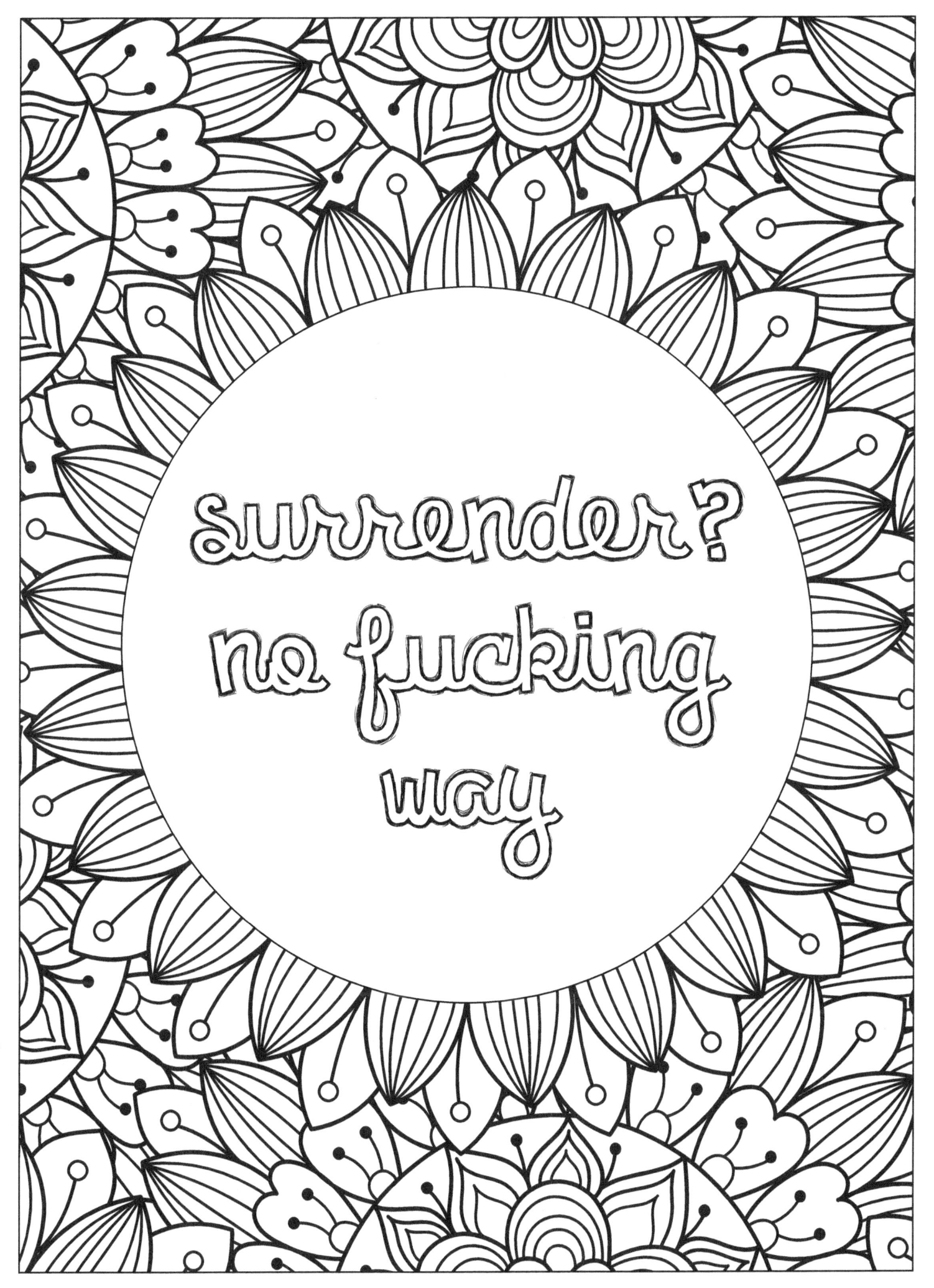

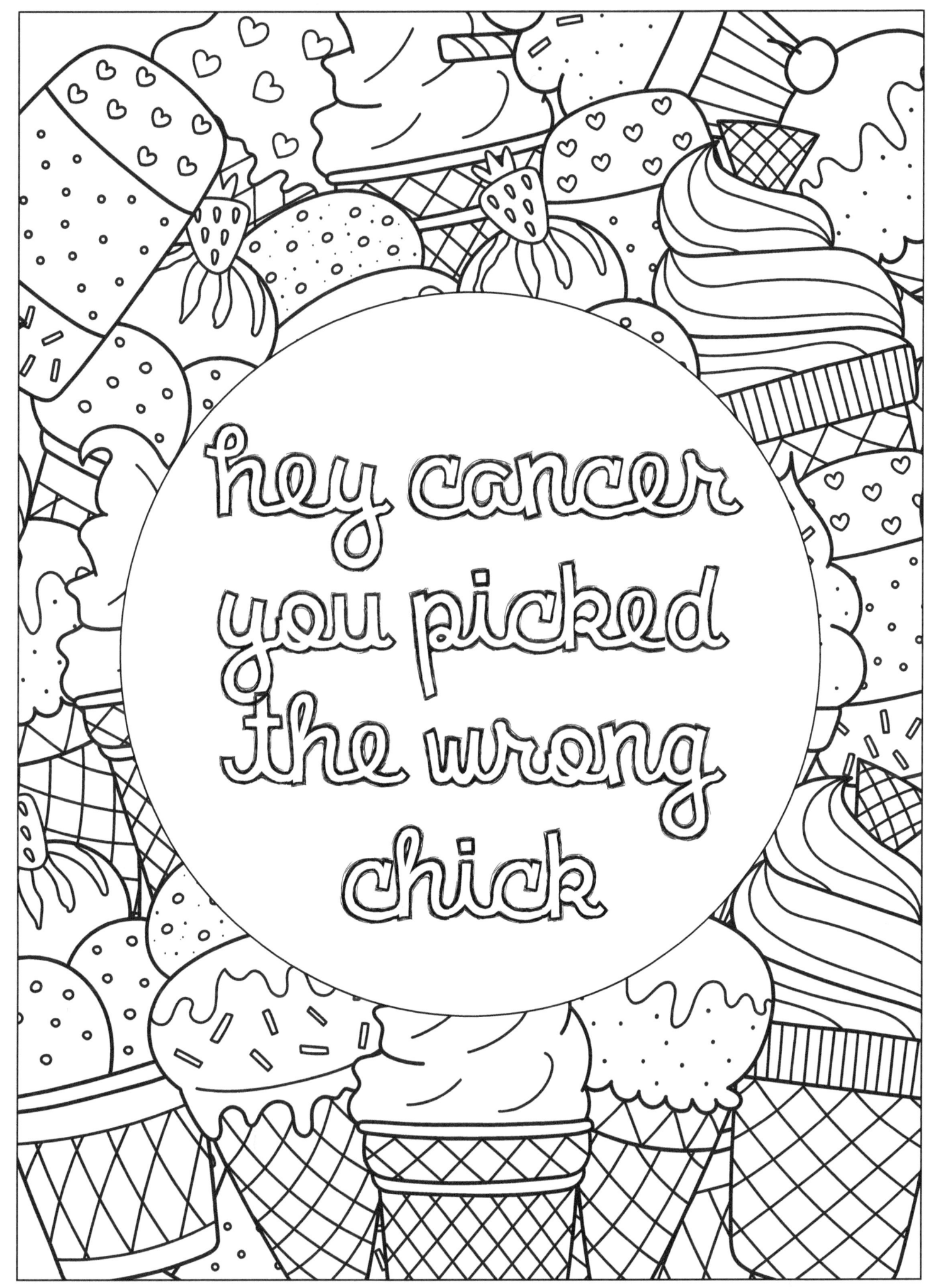

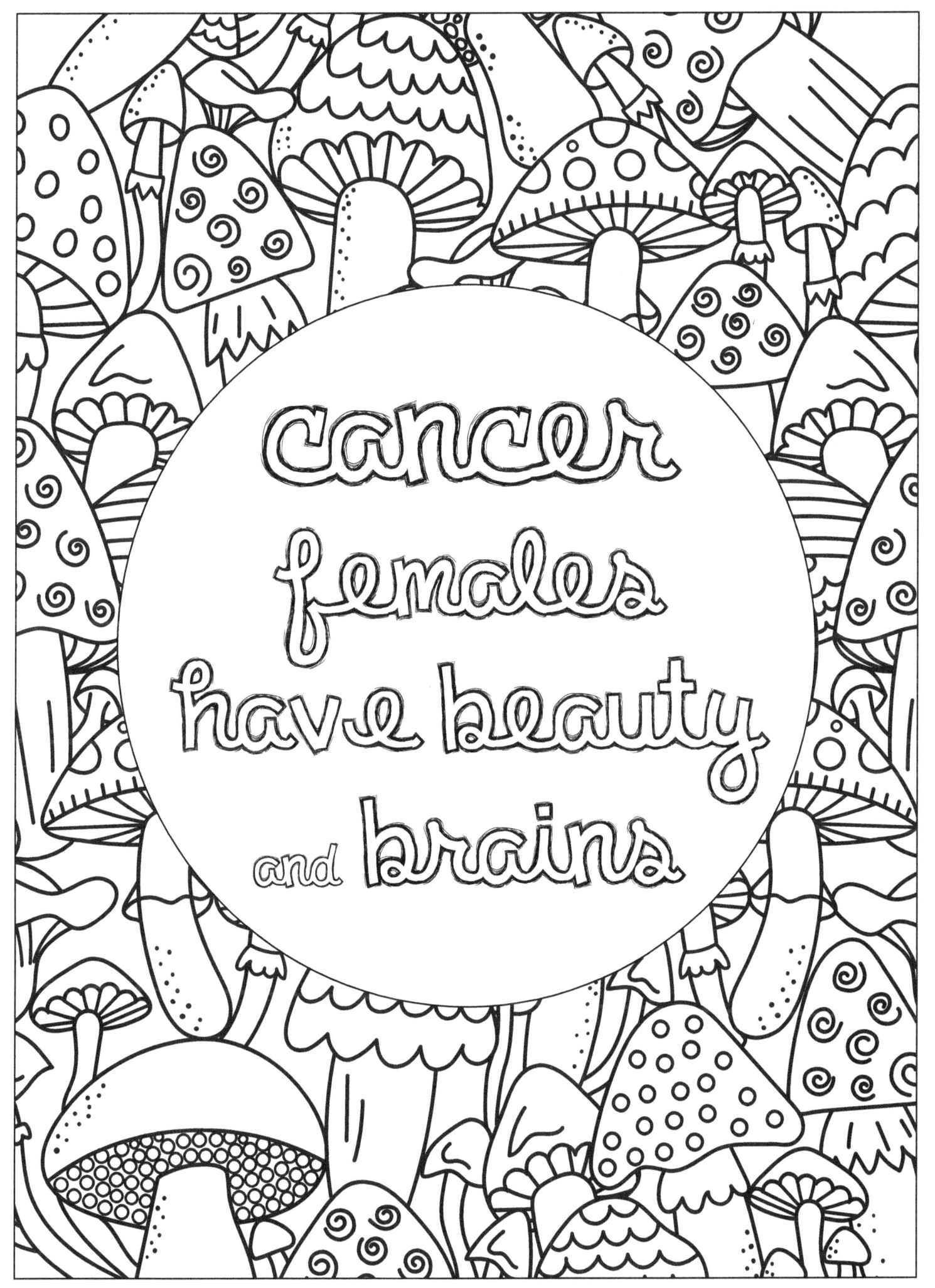

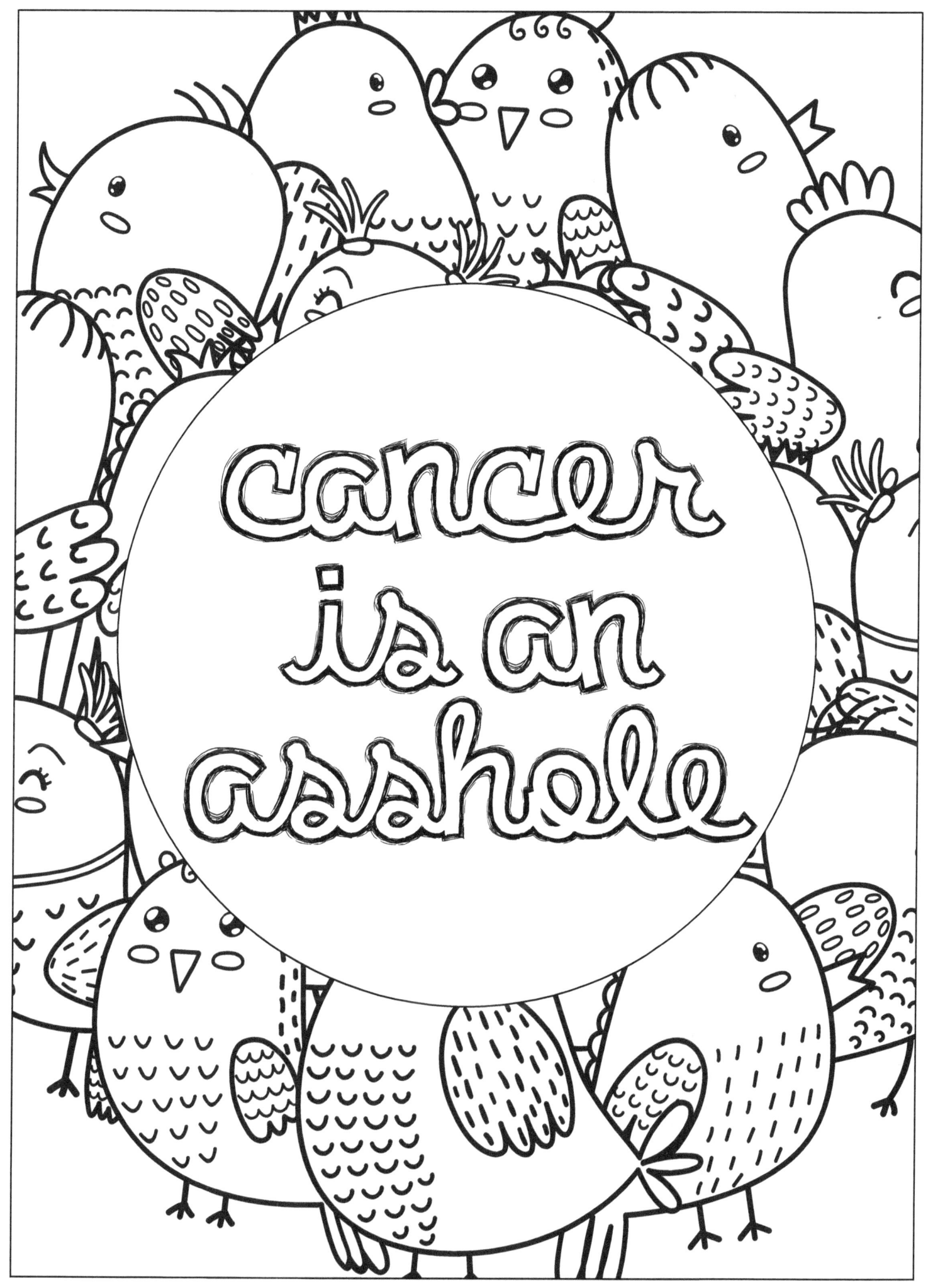

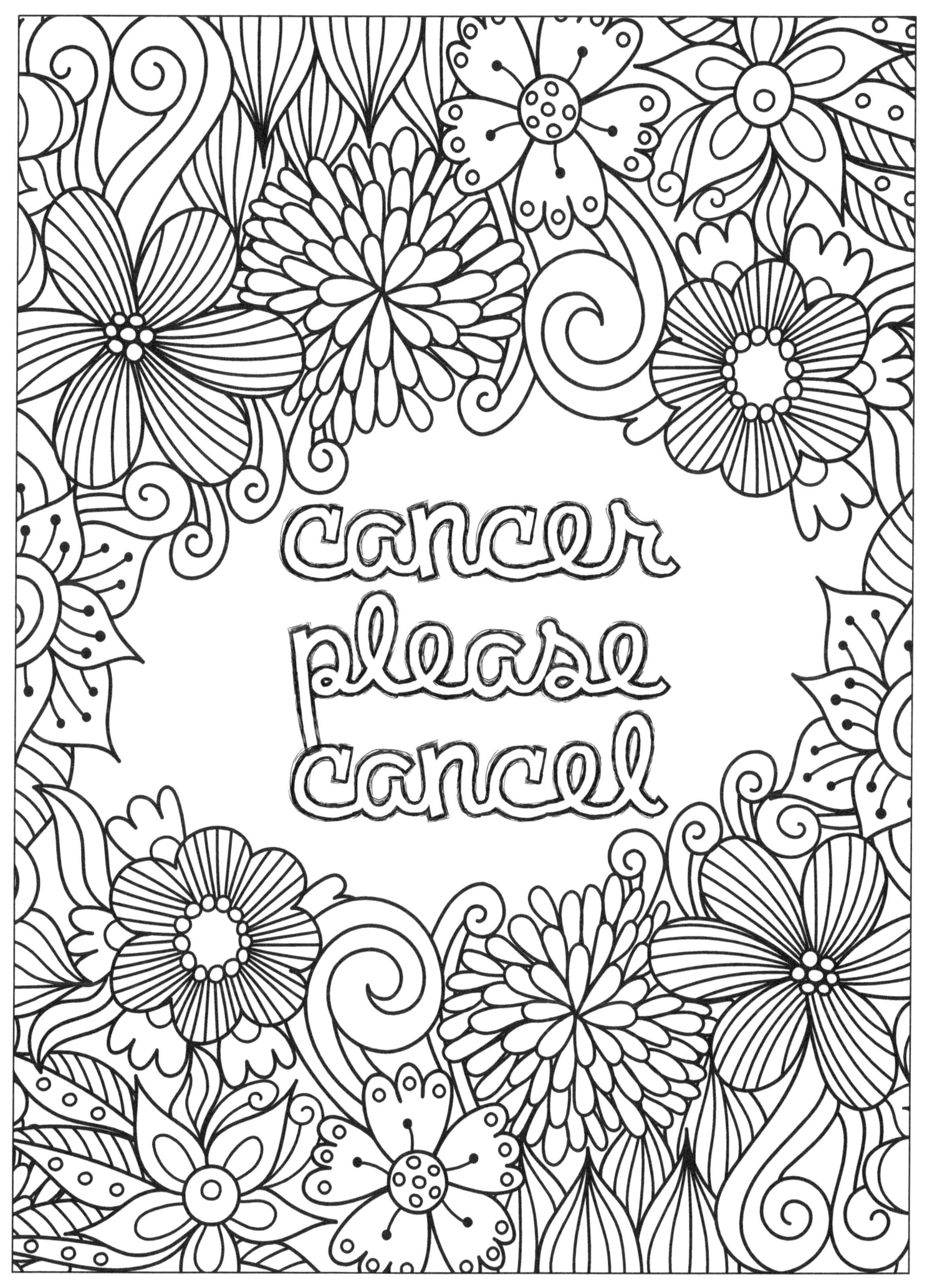

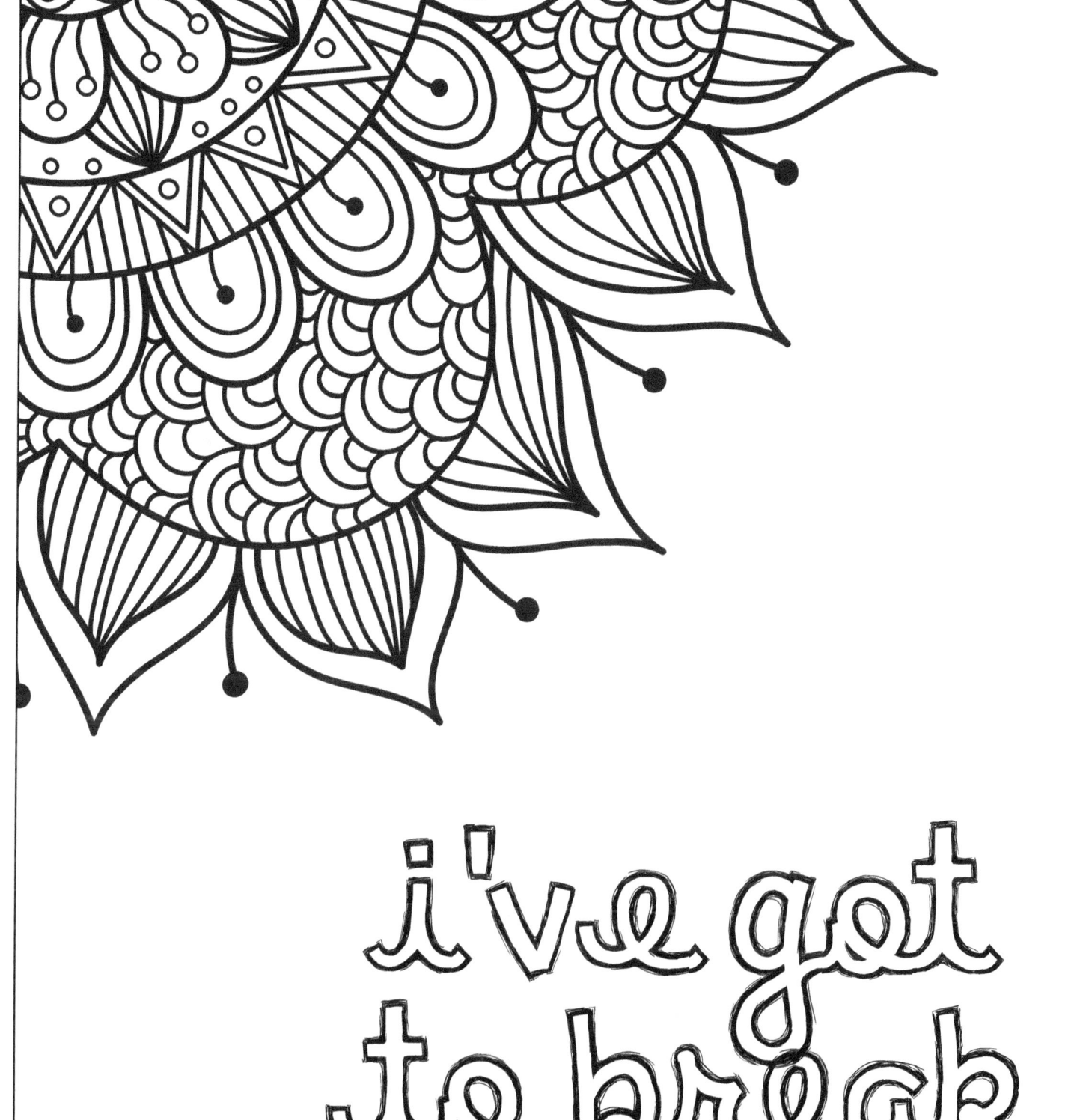

i've got
to break
free

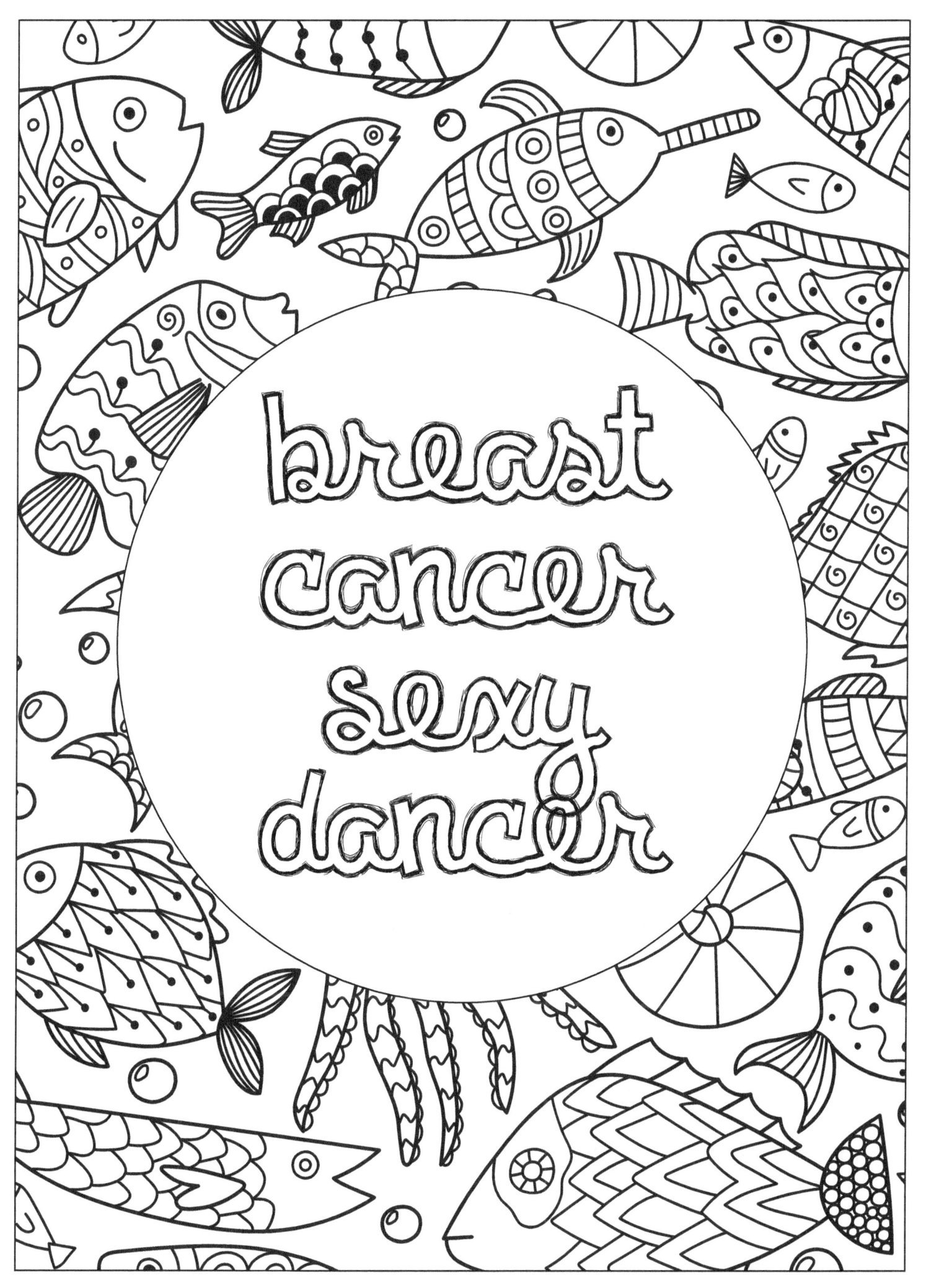

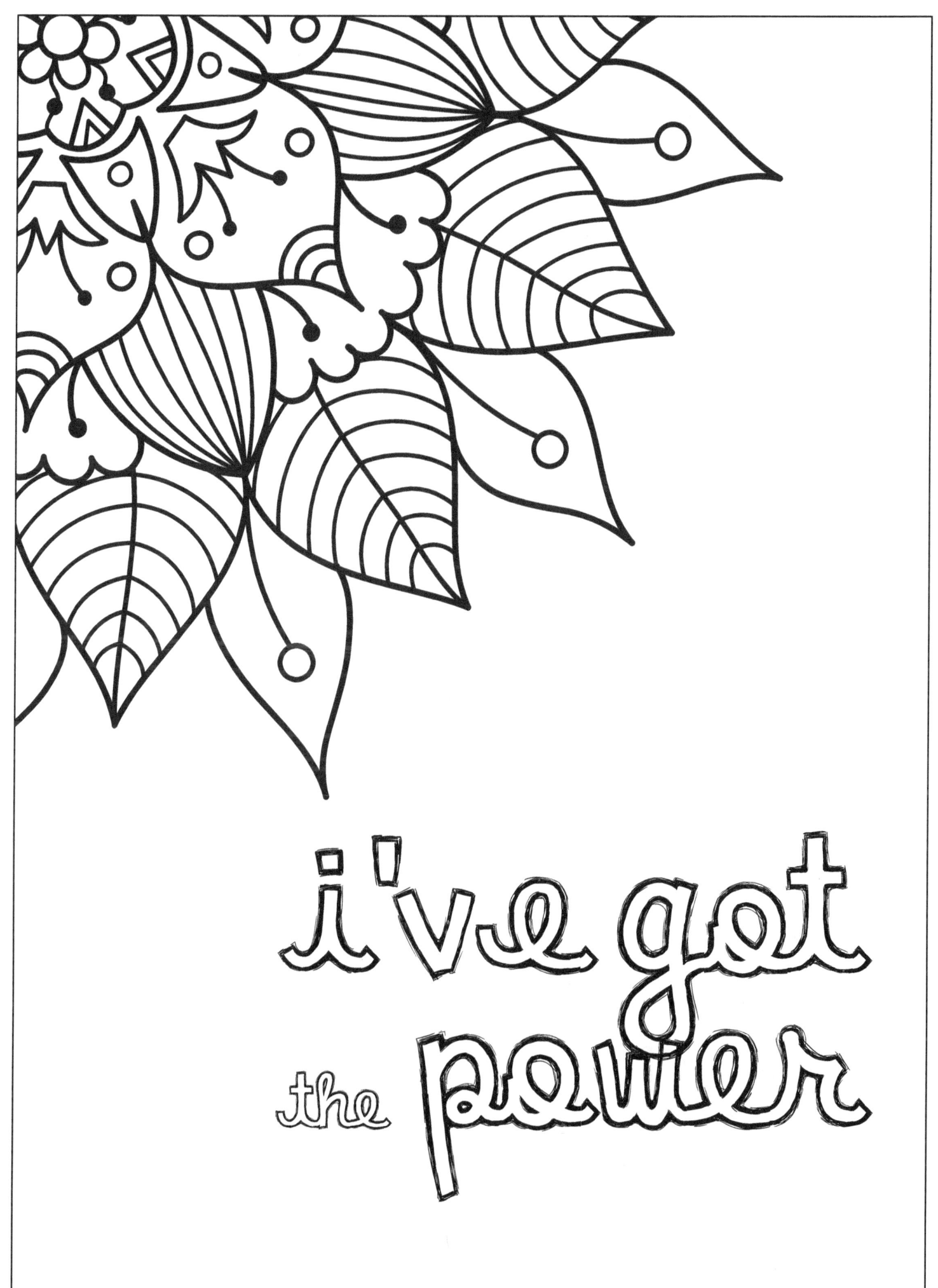

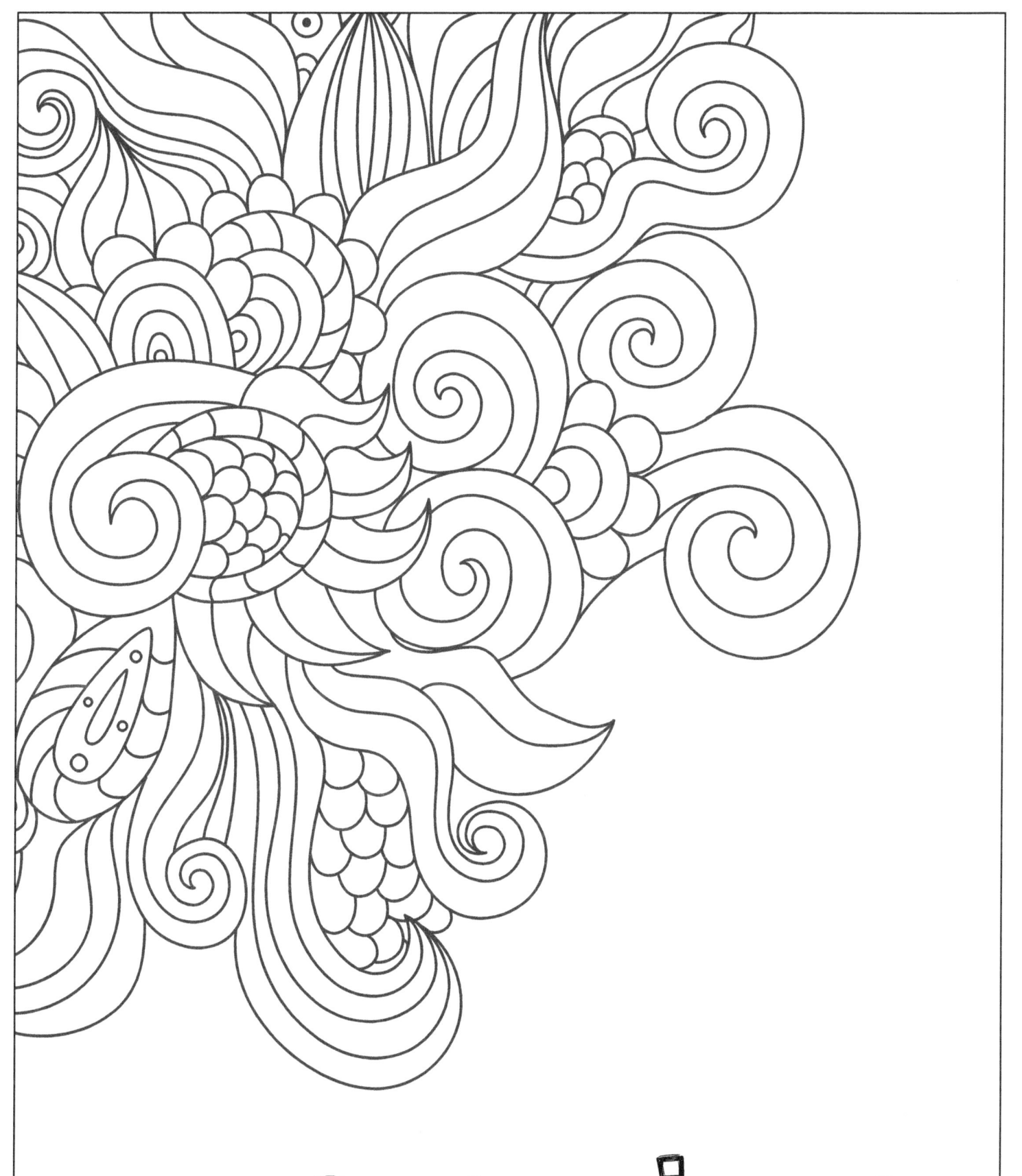

survivor

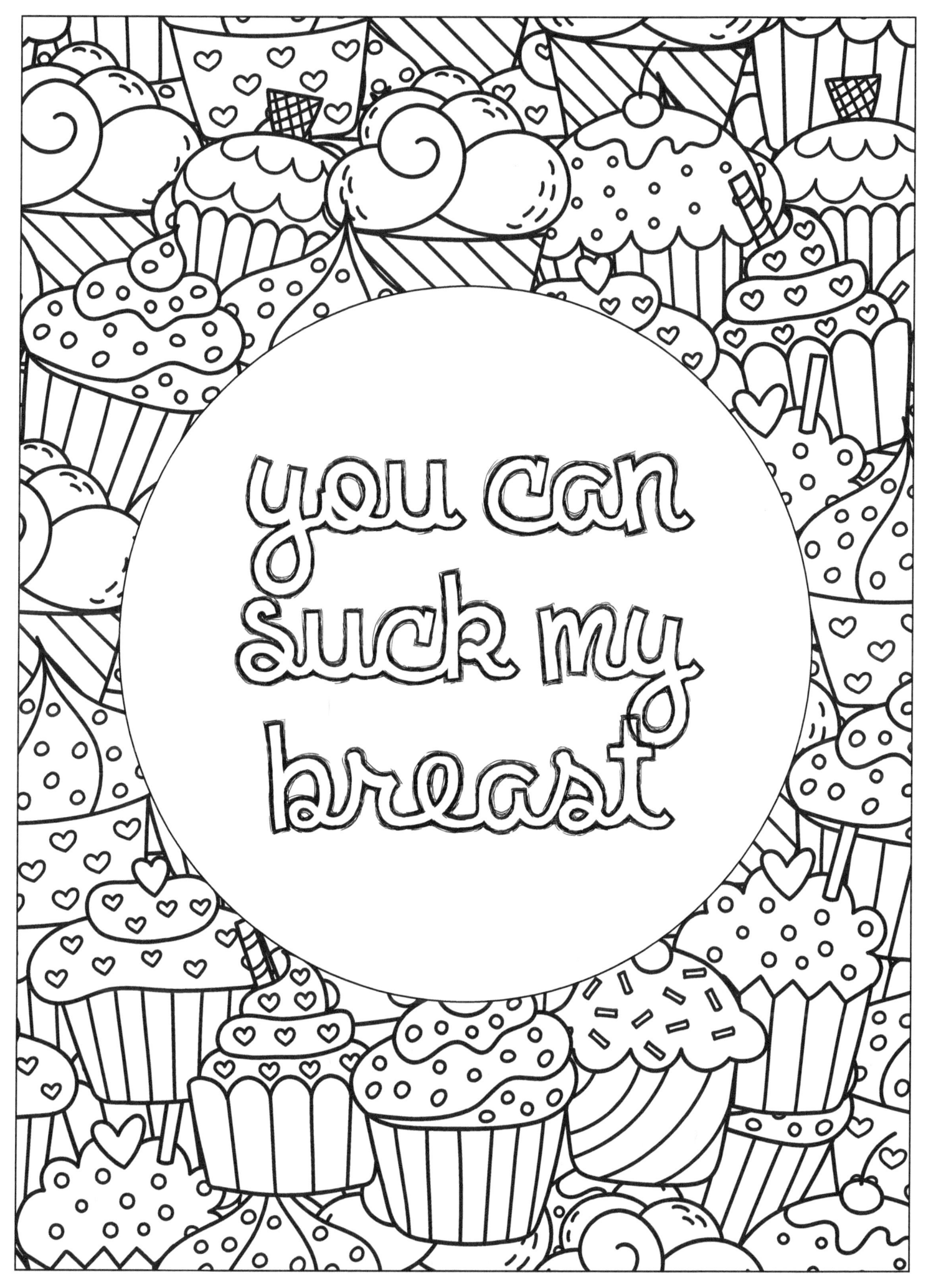

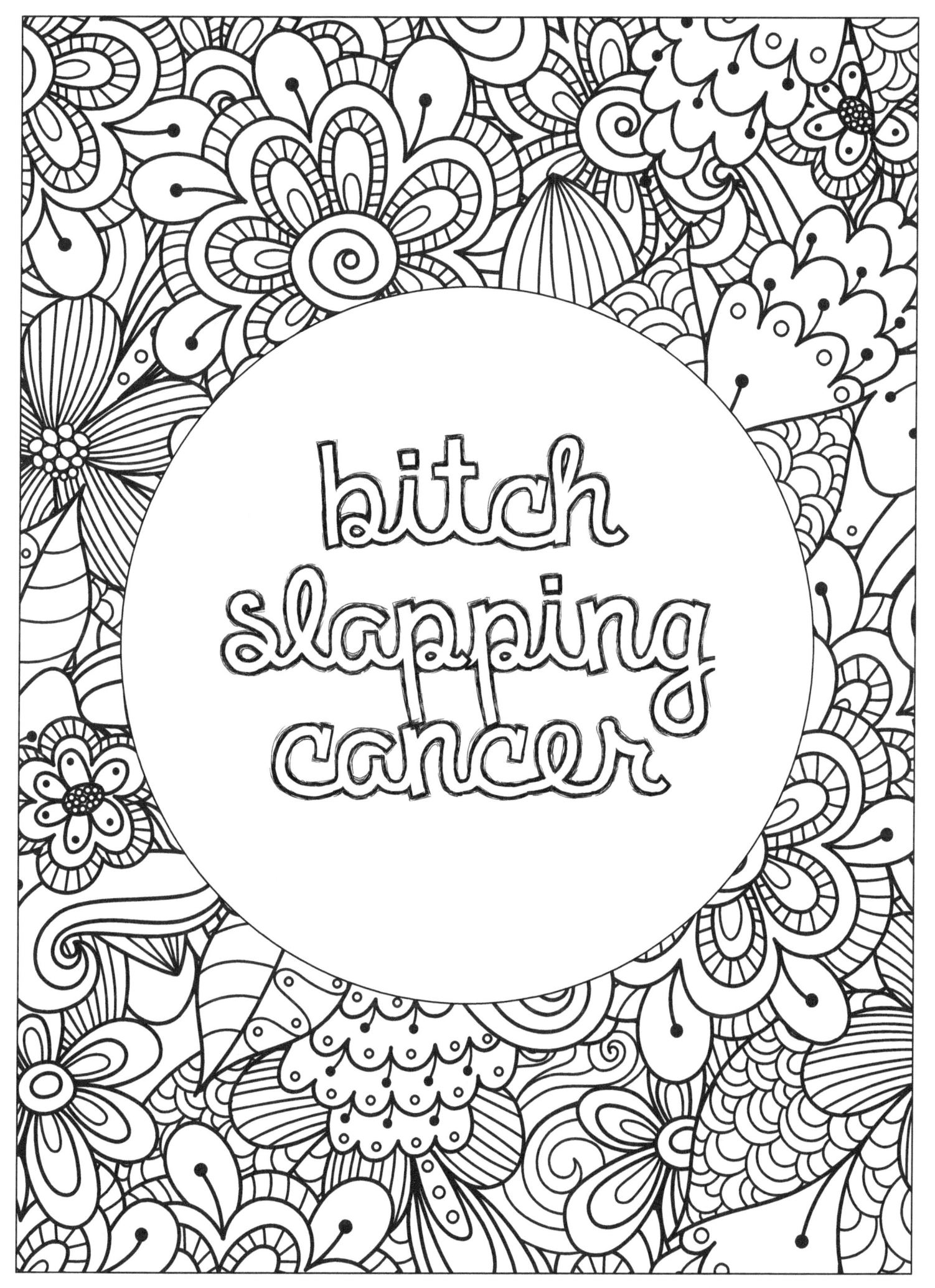

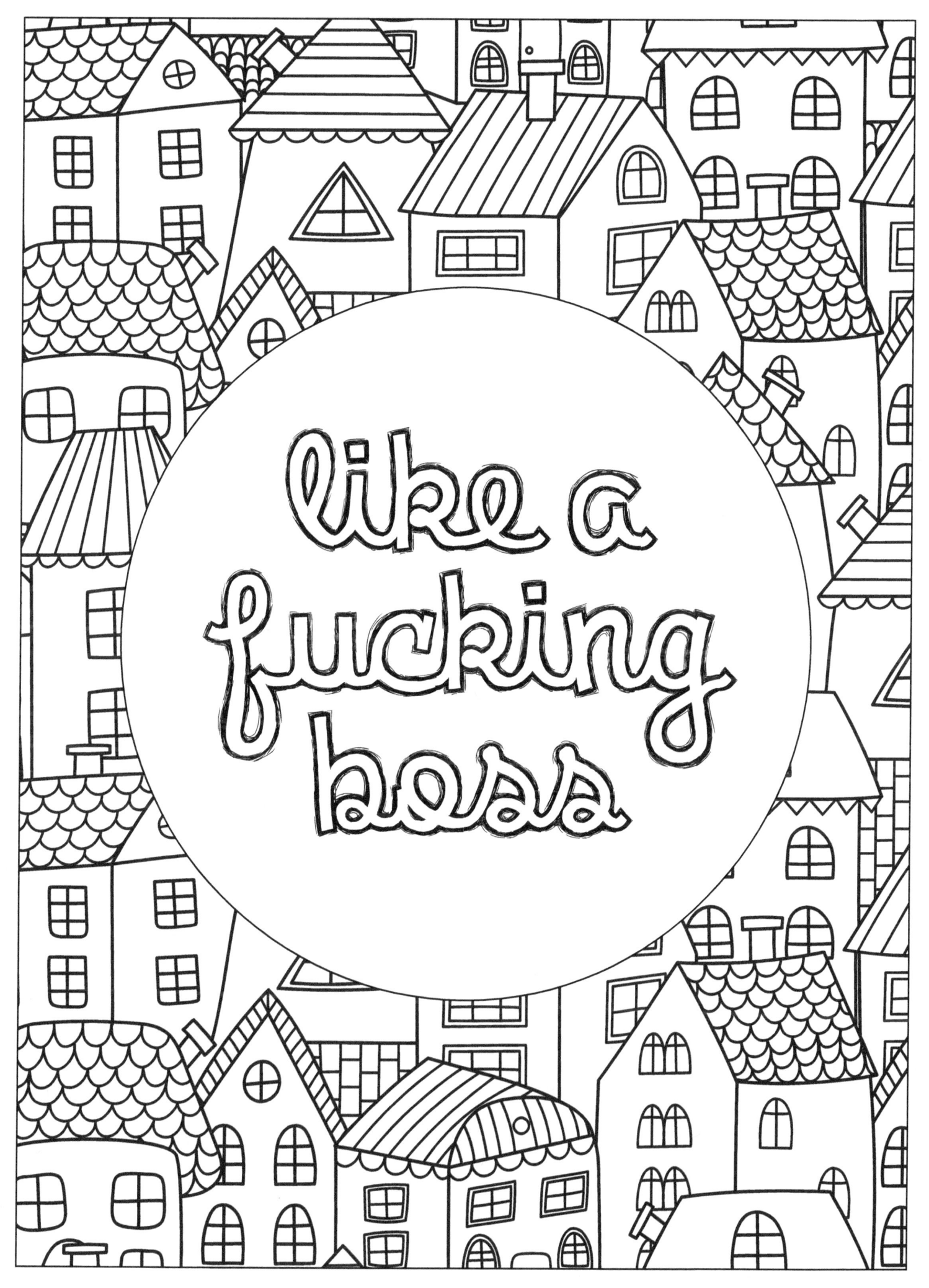

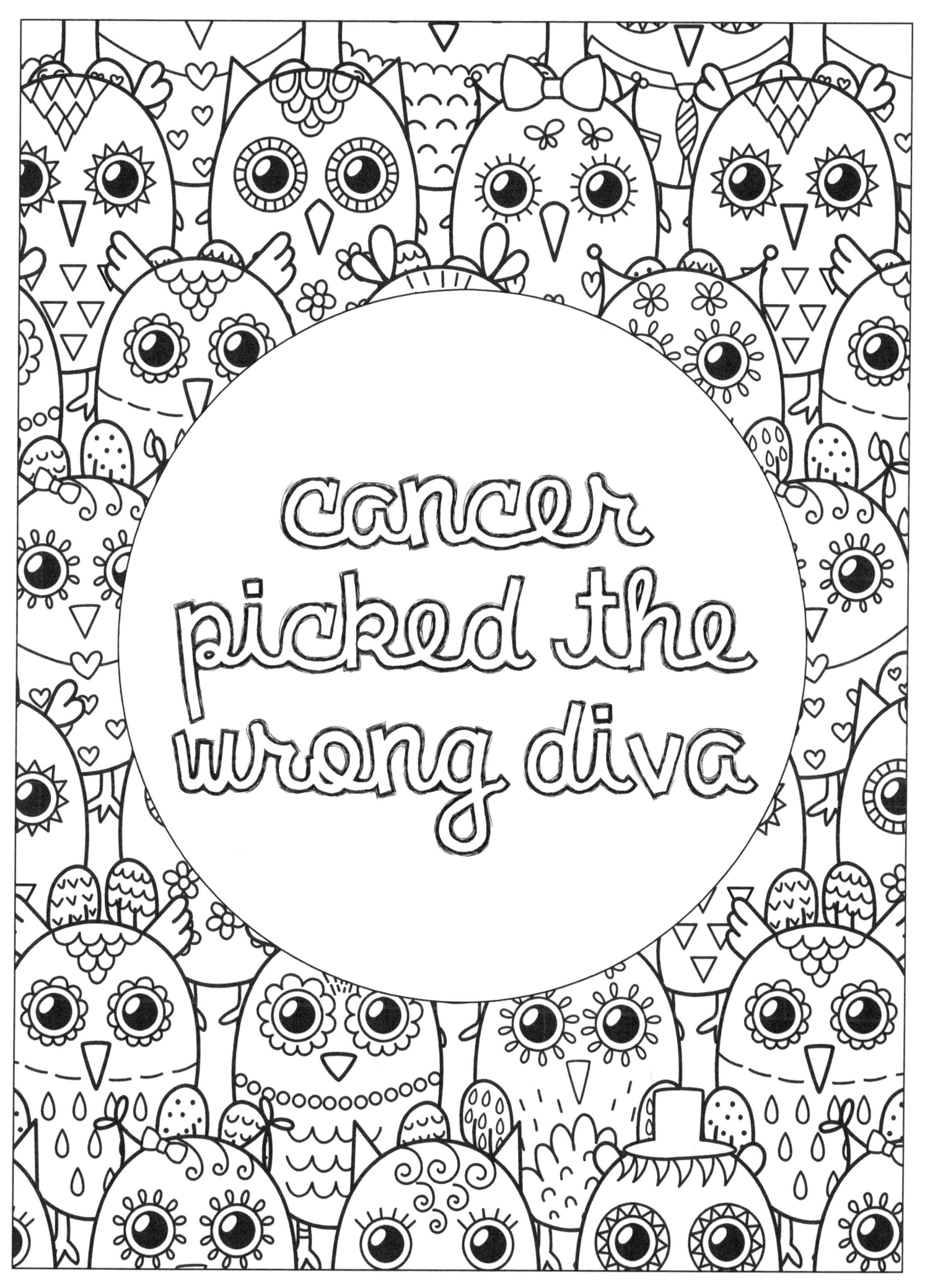

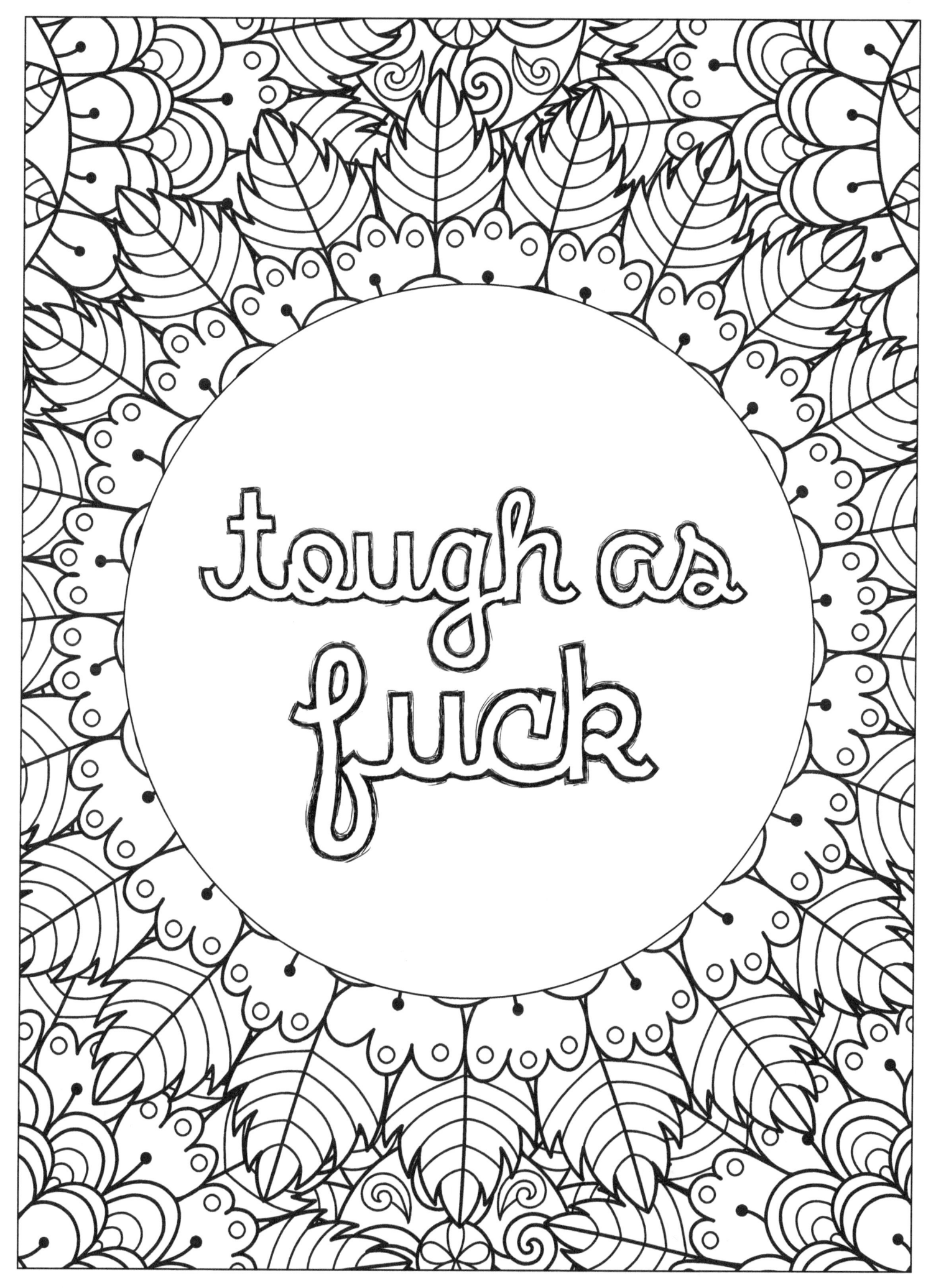

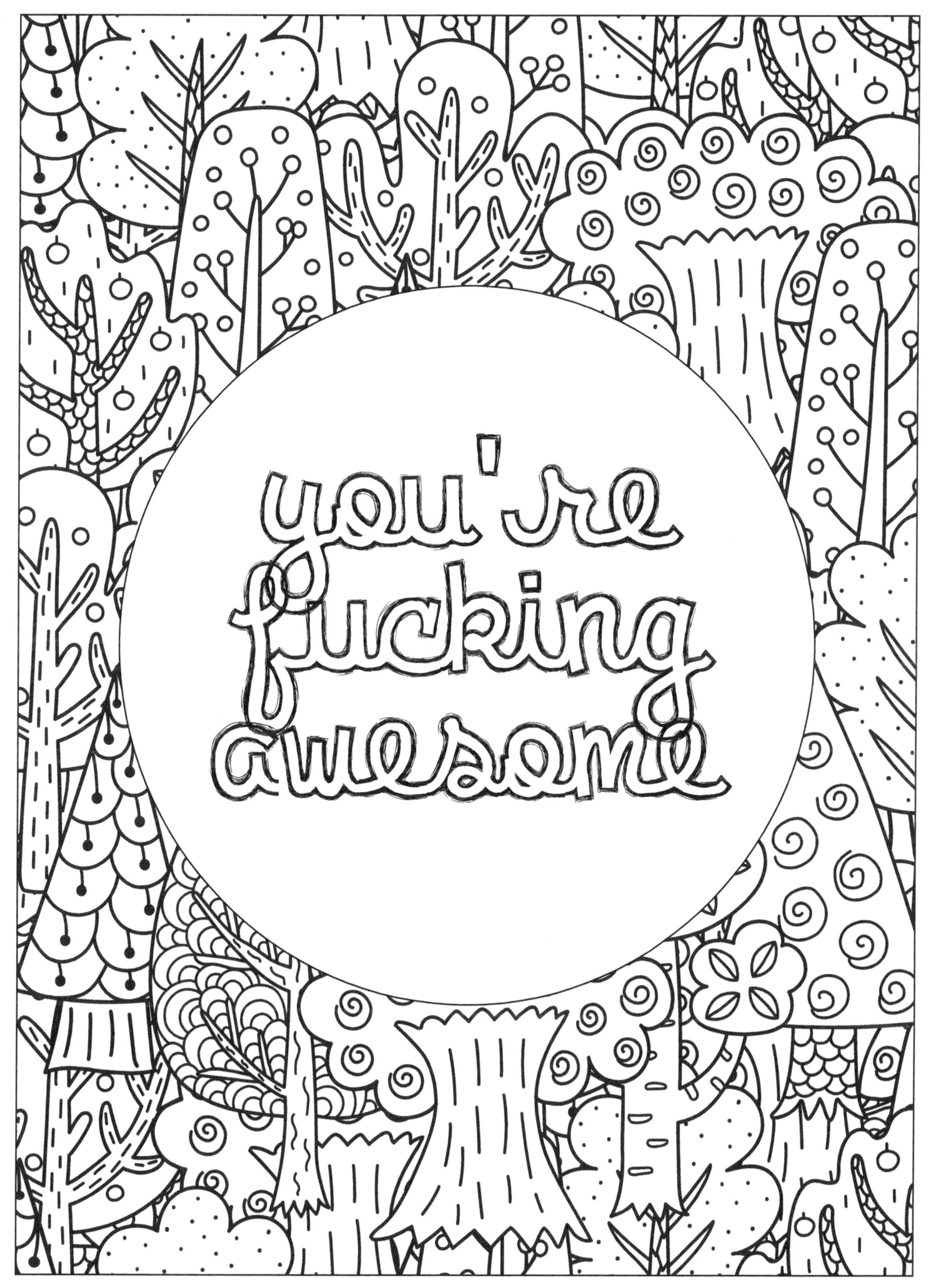

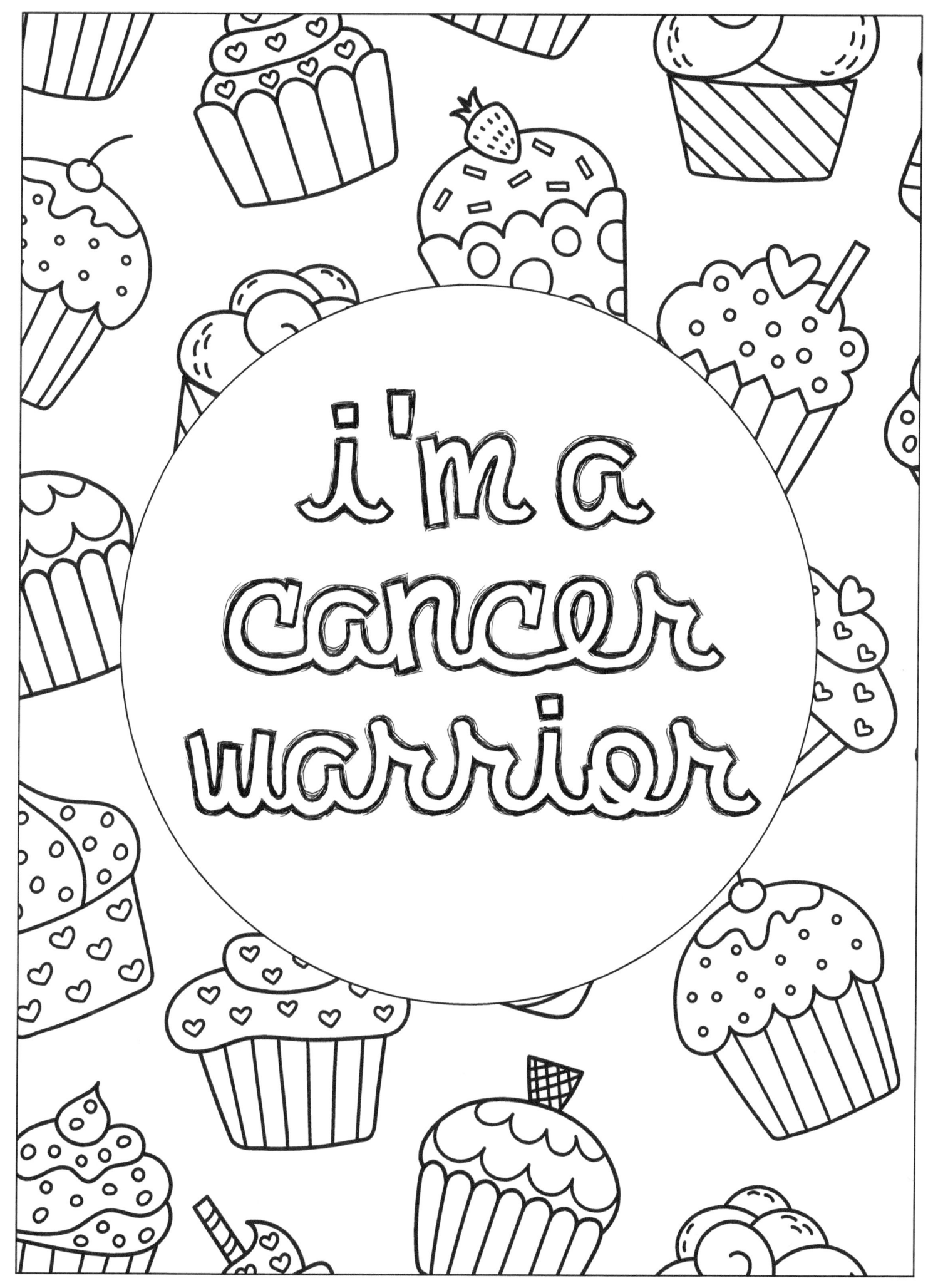

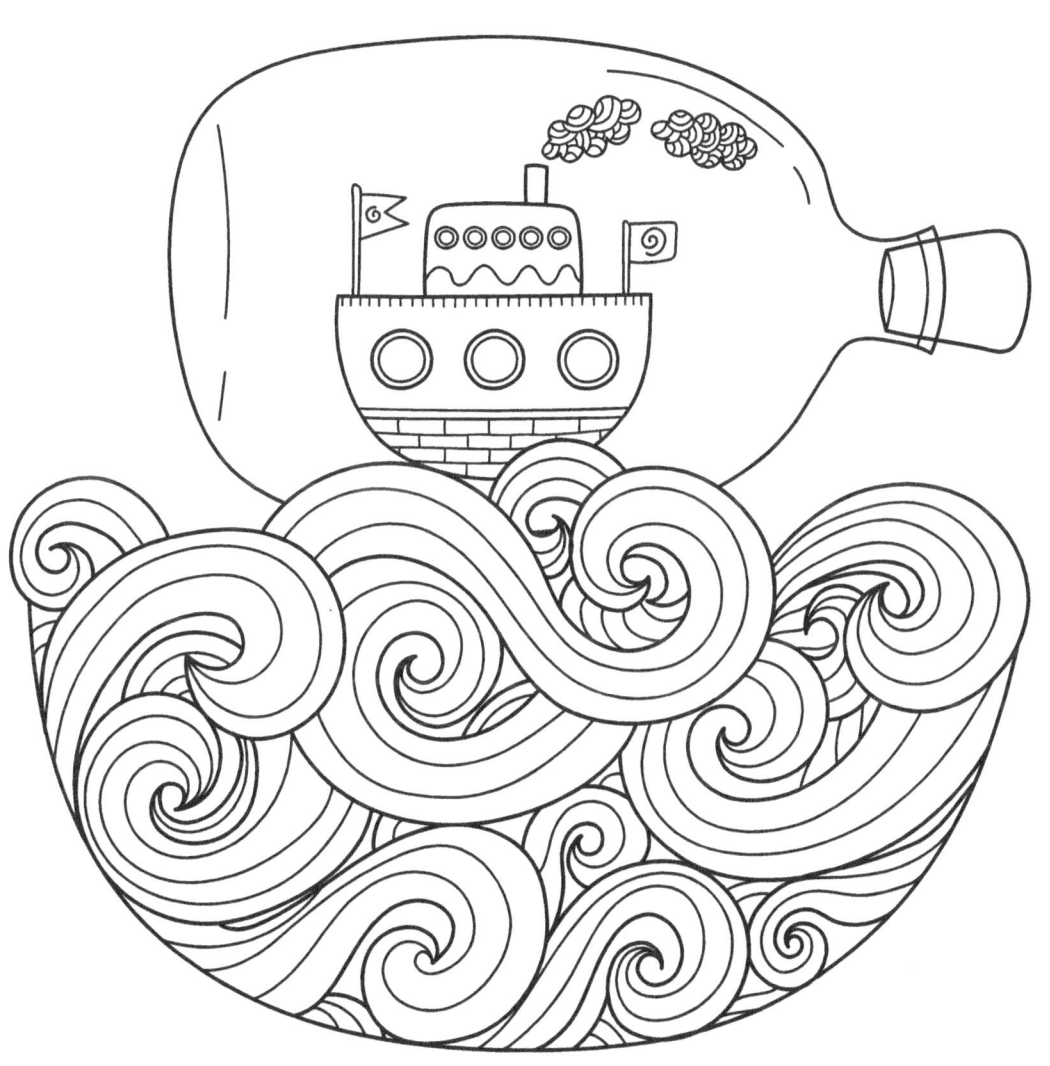

it's a long journey

but you are a true fighter

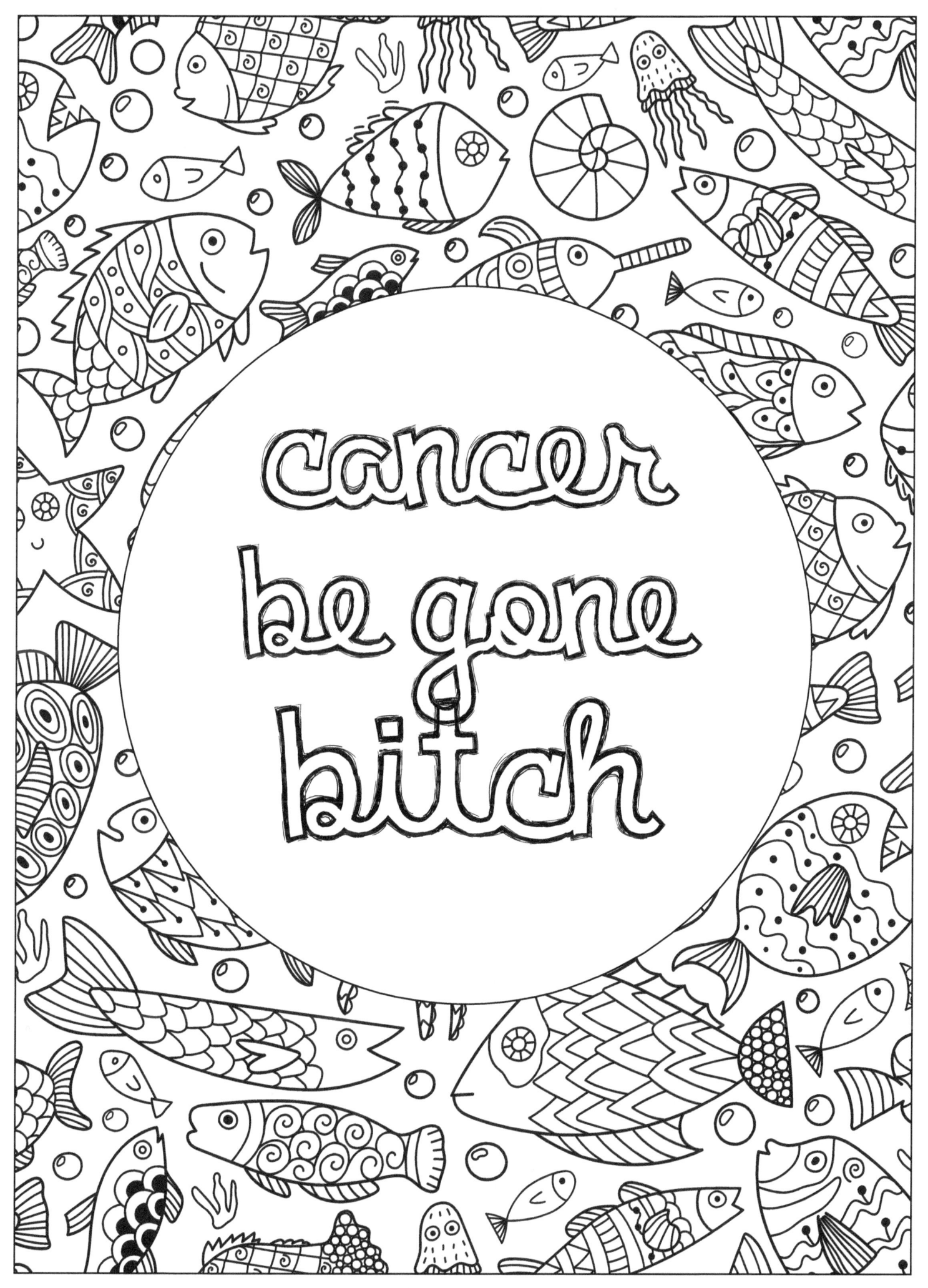

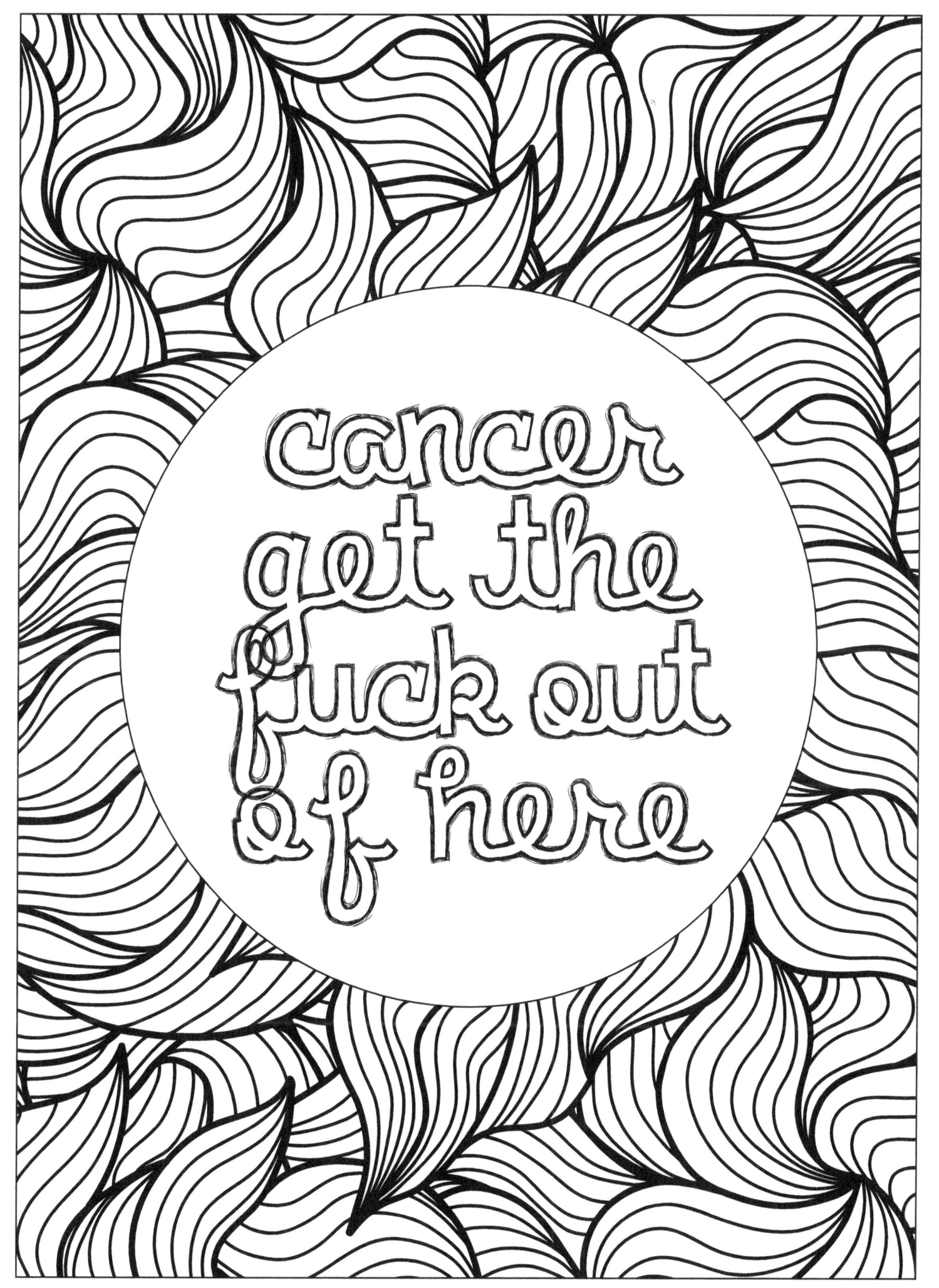

www.ingramcontent.com/pod-product-compliance
Lightning Source LLC
Chambersburg PA
CBHW080450290526

45791CB00008BA/2660